TRIVIA
SENIORS

INTRODUCTION

Welcome to "Trivia for Seniors"! This trivia book is a delightful journey through the past, tailor-made for seniors who cherish the memories of bygone eras. We invite you to embark on a nostalgic quest, rekindling the moments that have shaped our lives. As you turn the pages of this book, you'll revisit history and make new memories by challenging your knowledge and wit.

What to Expect?

Diverse Themes: Our trivia questions delve into various facets of the past, from unforgettable historical events to iconic pop culture moments. With 400 questions, you'll rediscover the magic of yesteryears.

Multiple Choices: Each question presents four possible answers (A, B, C, and D). Simply circle your chosen answer, and when you're ready, flip to the back of the book to unveil the correct responses.
Benefits of "Trivia for Seniors":

Memory Enhancement: Exercising your brain with trivia improves memory retention, cognitive function, and mental agility.

Entertainment: Enjoy hours of entertainment and relaxation with large-print questions and answers designed for easy reading.

So, are you ready to journey through the decades, testing your knowledge and savoring the moments that matter? Let's dive into "Trivia for Seniors"!

May this book bring joy, laughter, and a deeper connection to the wonderful tapestry of your life's adventures.

Happy Trivia Time!

TABLE OF CONTENTS

GET YOUR FREE E-BOOKS

➢ Scan QR Code

➢ Download E-Books

➢ Print and Start Boosting Your Brain

OR
go to our website

marywidkins.com

THE FABULOUS FIFTIES

1. Which popular toy was introduced in the 1950s?
a) Teddy bear
b) Rubik's Cube
c) Hula hoop
d) Action Man

2. Who was the U.S. President for most of the 1950s?
a) Harry S. Truman
b) Richard Nixon
c) Dwight D. Eisenhower
d) John F. Kennedy

3. What 1951 movie starred Vivien Leigh and Marlon Brando?
a) Rear Window
b) A Streetcar Named Desire
c) On the Waterfront
d) Sunset Boulevard

4. Which artist is known as the "King of Rock and Roll"?
a) Chuck Berry
b) Johnny Cash
c) Elvis Presley
d) Buddy Holly

5. In 1954, Roger Bannister achieved what sporting milestone?
a) Scored 100 goals in a soccer season
b) Swam the English Channel
c) Ran a mile in under four minutes
d) Won five gold medals in the Olympics

6. Which T.V. show, premiering in 1951, starred Lucille Ball?
a) The Twilight Zone
b) The Ed Sullivan Show
c) The Beverly Hillbillies
d) I Love Lucy

7. In 1953, Sir Edmund Hillary and Tenzing Norgay became the first to...?
a) Cross the Atlantic in a balloon
b) Climb Mount Everest
c) Sail around the world
d) Reach the South Pole

8. Which Disney theme park opened in 1955?
a) Disney World
b) Epcot
c) Disneyland
d) Disney's Hollywood Studios

9. Which of these car models became an icon of the 1950s?
a) Model T Ford
b) Volkswagen Beetle
c) Chevrolet Corvette
d) Honda Civic

10. Which novel, written by J.D. Salinger and published in 1951, became an immediate classic?
a) On the Road
b) To Kill a Mockingbird
c) Brave New World
d) The Catcher in the Rye

11. Which iconic actor starred as a troubled rebel in the 1955 film "Rebel Without a Cause"?
a) Marlon Brando
b) Paul Newman
c) James Dean
d) Cary Grant

12. Which groundbreaking 1950s T.V. show was set in New York and focused on a Cuban bandleader and his wife?
a) The Honeymooners
b) I Love Lucy
c) The Perry Como Show
d) The Jack Benny Program

13. Which of these was NOT a popular 1950s dance?
a) The Twist
b) The Jitterbug
c) The Mashed Potato
d) The Waltz

14. In which U.S. state was the first McDonald's restaurant opened in 1955?
a) California
b) Illinois
c) Texas
d) Florida

15. The 1954 Supreme Court case, Brown v. Board of Education, declared segregation in public schools as...?
a) Constitutional
b) Unconstitutional
c) A state's choice
d) A district's choice

16. Which classic 1950s sci-fi film featured an alien named Klaatu?
a) Invasion of the Body Snatchers
b) Forbidden Planet
c) The Day the Earth Stood Still
d) War of the Worlds

17. What type of music, rooted in African-American communities of New Orleans, gained immense popularity in the 1950s?
a) Swing
b) Jazz
c) Rock 'n' Roll
d) Blues

18. Which automobile company introduced the "Thunderbird" model in the 1950s?
a) Chevrolet
b) Chrysler
c) Ford
d) Dodge

19. Who famously said, "In the future, everyone will be world-famous for 15 minutes," during the 1950s?
a) Frank Sinatra
b) Marilyn Monroe
c) John F. Kennedy
d) Andy Warhol

20. Which actress starred alongside Humphrey Bogart in the 1951 film "The African Queen"?
a) Lauren Bacall
b) Audrey Hepburn
c) Katharine Hepburn
d) Bette Davis

21. Who was the original host of the 1950s quiz show "The $64,000 Question"?
a) Hal March
b) Jack Barry
c) Bill Cullen
d) Bob Barker

22. In which 1950s Alfred Hitchcock film set in San Francisco does a man become obsessed with his former lover?
a) Psycho
b) Rear Window
c) North by Northwest
d) Vertigo

23. Which crooner released the hit song "Mack the Knife" in the late 1950s?
a) Frank Sinatra
b) Bobby Darin
c) Perry Como
d) Dean Martin

24. In which fictional town is "The Andy Griffith Show" (1960) set?
a) Springfield
b) Mayfield
c) Hooterville
d) Mayberry

25. Which 1952 musical film features Gene Kelly's "Singin' in the Rain"?
a) An American in Paris
b) The Band Wagon
c) On the Town
d) Singin' in the Rain

26. Which 1957 film focuses on jurors discussing a defendant's reasonable doubt?
a) To Kill a Mockingbird
b) The Verdict
c) 12 Angry Men
d) Judgment at Nuremberg

27. To which U.S. President did Marilyn Monroe sing "Happy Birthday"?
a) Dwight D. Eisenhower
b) Richard Nixon
c) John F. Kennedy
d) Lyndon B. Johnson

28. Which 1955 Disney character declared, "Just remember what your old pal said: you've got a friend in me"?
a) Mickey Mouse
b) Donald Duck
c) Goofy
d) Trick question: it is from "Toy Story" (1995)

29. Which 1950s "Space Western" TV show was set in space?
a) Gunsmoke
b) Star Trek
c) The Twilight Zone
d) Space Patrol

30. Which 1950s musical duo debuted with "Bye Bye Love"?
a) Simon & Garfunkel
b) The Everly Brothers
c) Hall & Oates
d) Sonny & Cher

31. James Stewart and Kim Novak starred together in which hauntingly romantic 1958 Hitchcock film?
a) Rope
b) The Birds
c) Vertigo
d) Dial M for Murder

32. The game of "Risk," introduced in the 1950s, revolves around what central theme?
a) Real estate acquisition
b) Global domination
c) Murder mystery
d) Card trading

33. Which film featured Marlon Brando as Stanley Kowalski shouting, "Stella!"?
a) The Godfather
b) On the Waterfront
c) Guys and Dolls
d) A Streetcar Named Desire

34. "Rock Around the Clock" is a seminal rock and roll song from the 1950s by which artist?
a) Elvis Presley
b) Chuck Berry
c) Bill Haley & His Comets
d) Little Richard

35. Which popular board game introduced in the 1950s is about discovering an opponent's hidden fleet?
a) Clue
b) Battleship
c) Connect Four
d) Monopoly

36. Which iconic 1950s T.V. game show had contestants answering in the form of a question?
a) The Price Is Right
b) Jeopardy!
c) Who Wants to Be a Millionaire?
d) Wheel of Fortune

37. Which artist was a member of "The Quarrymen" in the 1950s before going solo?
a) Bob Dylan
b) Mick Jagger
c) Paul McCartney
d) Freddie Mercury

38. Which late 1950s film showcased the life of Roman slave Judah Ben-Hur?
a) Spartacus
b) Cleopatra
c) Gladiator
d) Ben-Hur

39. Which 1950s game had players touch colored circles on a mat with their bodies?
a) Charades
b) Twister
c) Pictionary
d) Simon Says

40. Which 1959 film took viewers on a suspenseful journey on the "North by Northwest" Orient Express?
a) Strangers on a Train
b) Vertigo
c) Rear Window
d) North by Northwest

41. Whose orchestra produced the 1950s hit "Mambo No. 5"?
a) Glenn Miller
b) Benny Goodman
c) Perez Prado
d) Duke Ellington

42. Which 1950s game involves players constructing crosswords for points?
a) Boggle
b) Jenga
c) Scrabble
d) Monopoly

43. What film featuring Charlton Heston was known for its spectacular chariot race scene?
a) Spartacus
b) The Ten Commandments
c) Gladiator
d) Ben-Hur

44. Which singer became known as the "Chairman of the Board" during the 1950s?
a) Frank Sinatra
b) Bing Crosby
c) Dean Martin
d) Tony Bennett

45. What is the central objective in the 1950s game "Mouse Trap"?
a) Collecting cheese
b) Building a mousetrap
c) Evading a cat
d) Trapping the opponent's mouse pieces

46. Which 1956 film made Elvis Presley a box office sensation?
a) Jailhouse Rock
b) Blue Hawaii
c) King Creole
d) Love Me Tender

47. Which musical style, characterized by its rapid rhythm, became popular in the 1950s and originated in Cuba?
a) Salsa
b) Mambo
c) Cha-cha-cha
d) Reggaeton

48. Which sci-fi movie, released in 1951, showcases an alien visitor and his robot, Gort?
a) The War of the Worlds
b) Forbidden Planet
c) The Day the Earth Stood Still
d) Invasion of the Body Snatchers

49. Which 1950s board game requires players to solve a murder mystery in a mansion?
a) Battleship
b) Risk
c) Clue (or Cluedo)
d) Life

50. Which 1952 film about Hollywood's shift from silent to talkies won eight Academy Awards?
a) Gone with the Wind
b) A Streetcar Named Desire
c) Singin' in the Rain
d) Casablanca

51. Who starred as the titular character in the 1953 film "Shane"?
a) James Stewart
b) Gregory Peck
c) Alan Ladd
d) Gary Cooper

52. Which 1950s toy is spun using a string and a wrist flick?
a) Slinky
b) Hula hoop
c) Yo-yo
d) Rubik's Cube

53. Which songstress had a hit with "Tennessee Waltz" in the early 1950s?
a) Ella Fitzgerald
b) Patsy Cline
c) Peggy Lee
d) Patti Page

54. Which 1956 movie depicts the biblical tale of Moses in ancient Egypt?
a) The Robe
b) Cleopatra
c) The Ten Commandments
d) Quo Vadis

55. In which game from the 1950s would players navigate their peg family in a car through various life events?
a) Operation
b) Monopoly
c) Life
d) Parcheesi

56. What U.S. state became the 50th to join the union in 1959?
a) Hawaii
b) Alaska
c) Arizona
d) New Mexico

57. Which author's 1957 novel "On the Road" epitomized the Beat Generation?
a) Jack Kerouac
b) F. Scott Fitzgerald
c) John Steinbeck
d) Ernest Hemingway

58. The 1950s saw the rise of which fast-food restaurant chain, known for its golden arches?
a) Burger King
b) Wendy's
c) K.F.C.
d) McDonald's

59. What iconic children's toy was introduced in 1959 and became one of the best-selling toys ever?
a) G.I. Joe
b) Slinky
c) Barbie Doll
d) Etch A Sketch

60. Which 1927 Atlantic solo pilot gained notoriety again in the 1950s?
a) Howard Hughes
b) Amelia Earhart
c) Charles Lindbergh
d) Richard Byrd

61. What was the primary material used in constructing the first satellite, Sputnik, launched by the USSR in 1957?
a) Titanium
b) Aluminum
c) Steel
d) Carbon Fiber

62. Who became the 34th President of the United States in 1953?
a) John F. Kennedy
b) Harry S. Truman
c) Dwight D. Eisenhower
d) Richard Nixon

63. Which horse-named Ford car, launched in 1964, echoed '50s popularity?
a) Thunderbird
b) Corvette
c) Mustang
d) Pinto

64. Which children's program featuring a lady with a magic mirror premiered on C.B.S. in 1955?
a) Sesame Street
b) The Mickey Mouse Club
c) Romper Room
d) Captain Kangaroo

65. Which 1950s kitchen appliance sped up meal preparation?
a) Electric can opener
b) Microwave oven
c) Food processor
d) Electric griddle

66. Which 1950s fashion trend, championed by Audrey Hepburn, showcased flared long skirts?
a) Mini skirt
b) Poodle skirt
c) A-line skirt
d) Pencil skirt

67. Which famed baseball player, known as the "Say Hey Kid," began his Major League career in the 1950s?
a) Mickey Mantle
b) Babe Ruth
c) Jackie Robinson
d) Willie Mays

68. The polio vaccine was developed in the 1950s by which physician?
a) Edward Jenner
b) Albert Sabin
c) Jonas Salk
d) Alexander Fleming

69. Which iconic film actress starred in the 1955 movie "The Seven Year Itch," featuring a scene with her white dress billowing?
a) Grace Kelly
b) Audrey Hepburn
c) Elizabeth Taylor
d) Marilyn Monroe

70. Which music genre, known for its rhythm, surged in popularity among 1950s youth?
a) Swing
b) Jazz
c) Rock 'n' Roll
d) Country

71. What 1950s kitchen gadget, allowed for the easy preparation of instant coffee?
a) Electric kettle
b) Coffee grinder
c) Percolator
d) French press

72. Which '50s technology transformed household news and entertainment?
a) Color television
b) Radio
c) Cassette tapes
d) VCR

73. Which '50s accessory added volume to women's skirts?
a) Stiletto heels
b) Poodle skirts
c) Petticoats
d) Pearls

74. Which iconic actor was known as the "King of Cool" and starred in movies like "The Blob" and "The Great Escape"?
a) James Dean
b) Steve McQueen
c) Paul Newman
d) Cary Grant

75. Which 1950s T.V. show featured a redhead named Lucy and her husband, Ricky?
a) The Donna Reed Show
b) Father Knows Best
c) The Dick Van Dyke Show
d) I Love Lucy

76. In which country did the 1952 revolution lead to the establishment of a republic?
a) Iran
b) Egypt
c) India
d) Greece

77. Who wrote the dystopian novel "Fahrenheit 451", published in 1953?
a) Aldous Huxley
b) Ray Bradbury
c) George Orwell
d) Kurt Vonnegut

78. Which '50s men's hairstyle featured hair combed back from the forehead?
a) Mohawk
b) Pompadour
c) Buzz cut
d) Afro

79. Which 1950s dance became widely popular and was named after a bird?
a) Jitterbug
b) Twist
c) Chicken Dance
d) Turkey Trot

80. The 1957 novel "On the Road" by Jack Kerouac became an influential work for which American subculture?
a) The Beatniks
b) The Hippies
c) The Punk movement
d) The Goths

THE SWINGING SIXTIES

81. Which band released the groundbreaking album "Sgt. Pepper's Lonely Hearts Club Band" in 1967?

a) The Rolling Stones
b) The Beatles
c) The Doors
d) The Beach Boys

82. Which 1965 musical features a governess for seven children and an aspiring nun?
a) Cabaret
b) West Side Story
c) The Sound of Music
d) Fiddler on the Roof

83. What game, popularized in the 1960s, involves stacking wooden blocks and trying not to topple the tower?
a) Twister
b) Jenga
c) Connect Four
d) KerPlunk

84. Who played the titular character in the 1961 film adaptation of "Breakfast at Tiffany's"?
a) Audrey Hepburn
b) Marilyn Monroe
c) Julie Andrews
d) Elizabeth Taylor

85. In 1964, which British group achieved success with the track "House of the Rising Sun"?
a) The Who
b) The Animals
c) The Kinks
d) The Yardbirds

86. Which game, launched in the 1960s, uses a thin black mat and requires players to place hands and feet on colored circles?
a) Simon
b) Operation
c) Twister
d) Pictionary

87. Which 1960s artist sang "What's New Pussycat?" and "It's Not Unusual"?
a) Tom Jones
b) Roy Orbison
c) Frank Sinatra
d) Engelbert Humperdinck

88. In which region is the 1962 film "Lawrence of Arabia" set?
a) Sub-Saharan Africa
b) South America
c) The Middle East
d) South Asia

89. In which 1960s board game do players acquire properties and charge others rent?
a) Risk
b) Scrabble
c) Monopoly
d) Clue

90. "The Good, the Bad, and the Ugly" (1966) is an iconic film from which movie genre?
a) Romantic Comedy
b) Horror
c) Spaghetti Western
d) Musical

91. Which Motown group had hits in the 1960s with "Stop! In the Name of Love" and "You Can't Hurry Love"?
a) The Supremes
b) The Temptations
c) The Four Tops
d) The Marvelettes

92. Which 1960s toy, known for its catchy jingle, is a long, tubular hoop twirled around the waist?
a) Frisbee
b) Hula Hoop
c) Skip-It
d) Slinky

93. Who played the iconic British secret agent James Bond in the 1964 film "Goldfinger"?
a) Sean Connery
b) Roger Moore
c) Pierce Brosnan
d) Timothy Dalton

94. Which 1960s band sang "Light My Fire" and "Riders on the Storm"?
a) The Doors
b) The Byrds
c) The Zombies
d) The Velvet Underground

95. Which 1960s game lets players "operate" on Cavity Sam?
a) Life
b) Operation
c) Guess Who?
d) Hungry Hungry Hippos

96. The 1967 film "The Graduate" features which actor in the lead role of Benjamin Braddock?
a) Dustin Hoffman
b) Jack Nicholson
c) Robert Redford
d) Paul Newman

97. Which song by The Beach Boys, released in 1966, describes an idyllic and harmonious world?
a) California Girls
b) Good Vibrations
c) Surfin' U.S.A.
d) God Only Knows

98. What 1960s board game requires players to deduce which character committed a crime, with what weapon, and where?
a) Guess Who?
b) Battleship
c) Clue
d) Life

99. Who won the Best Actress Oscar in 1961 for her role in "Breakfast at Tiffany's"?
a) Audrey Hepburn
b) Julie Andrews
c) Elizabeth Taylor
d) Sophia Loren

100. In 1969, which event saw the first humans land on the moon?
a) Mercury Mission
b) Sputnik Launch
c) Gemini Project
d) Apollo 11 Mission

101. Which 1960 Alfred Hitchcock film is famous for its shocking shower scene?
a) Vertigo
b) Rear Window
c) The Birds
d) Psycho

102. Which 1969 event is seen as the peak of the hippie movement?
a) Monterey Pop Festival
b) Woodstock
c) Altamont Free Concert
d) Isle of Wight Festival

103. The 1960s miniskirt is most associated with which British fashion designer?
a) Vivienne Westwood
b) Stella McCartney
c) Mary Quant
d) Alexander McQueen

104. In 1967, which city experienced the "Summer of Love," attracting thousands of young people?
a) Los Angeles
b) New York
c) San Francisco
d) Chicago

105. Which 1962 novel by Ken Kesey features characters named Chief Bromden and Nurse Ratched?
a) Catch-22
b) Slaughterhouse-Five
c) One Flew Over the Cuckoo's Nest
d) The Electric Kool-Aid Acid Test

106. The 1964 Civil Rights Act aimed to end segregation in which country?
a) Canada
b) South Africa
c) United Kingdom
d) United States

107. Which toy, first introduced in the 1960s, allowed kids to create art by placing small colored pegs in a lit board?
a) Etch A Sketch
b) Spirograph
c) Lite-Brite
d) Colorforms

108. Which British band released the hit song "Paint It Black" in 1966?
a) The Rolling Stones
b) The Beatles
c) The Kinks
d) The Who

109. Which popular 1960s dance involved dancers making a "twisting" motion with their hips?
a) The Jive
b) The Mashed Potato
c) The Shimmy
d) The Twist

110. Which U.S. president declared the "War on Poverty" in the 1960s?
a) John F. Kennedy
b) Lyndon B. Johnson
c) Richard Nixon
d) Dwight D. Eisenhower

111. The 1966 World Cup was won by which country?
a) Brazil
b) Argentina
c) England
d) Germany

112. Which 1960s T.V. show featured the crew of the Starship Enterprise?
a) Star Wars: The Series
b) Doctor Who
c) Star Trek
d) Lost in Space

113. The 1960s show "The Flintstones" was set in which fictional prehistoric town?
a) Cavetown
b) Stoneville
c) Rockburg
d) Bedrock

114. Which 1963 speech famously declared, "I have a dream"?
a) Robert F. Kennedy's "Ripple of Hope"
b) Winston Churchill's "Iron Curtain"
c) Martin Luther King Jr.'s March on Washington speech
d) John F. Kennedy's "Moon" speech

115. Which 1960s hairstyle, also a bird's name, became popular and was notably worn by celebrities like Audrey Hepburn?
a) The Swan
b) The Pigeon
c) The Peacock
d) The Pixie

116. Which 1965 musical film features the von Trapp family singing in the Austrian Alps?
a) Mary Poppins
b) My Fair Lady
c) The Sound of Music
d) West Side Story

117. Which band had a 1966 hit with the song "Good Vibrations"?
a) The Monkees
b) The Beach Boys
c) The Byrds
d) The Turtles

118. The feminist movement of the 1960s was inspired in part by which 1963 book by Betty Friedan?
a) The Second Sex
b) Women, Culture, and Society
c) Sexual Politics
d) The Feminine Mystique

119. Which classic 1960s toy, a colorful face-changing puzzle, has become an iconic symbol of the decade?
a) Rubik's Cube
b) Magic 8 Ball
c) Tamagotchi
d) Troll dolls

120. In 1967, the Beatles sang "All You Need Is..." what?
a) Peace
b) Time
c) Love
d) Dreams

121. Which 1960s dance craze involves swaying your hips and moving your hands in a circular motion?
a) The Jitterbug
b) The Hula-Hoop
c) The Loco-motion
d) The Watusi

122. Which 1960s animated series follows the futuristic life of a family in the 21st century?
a) The Flintstones
b) The Jetsons
c) Scooby-Doo
d) Tom and Jerry

123. Which 1960s musical features a magical nanny in London?
a) Chitty Chitty Bang Bang
b) The Wizard of Oz
c) Mary Poppins
d) Annie

124. What popular 1960s fashion item was named after a French atomic bomb testing site due to its "explosive" effect on the viewer?
a) Poncho
b) Bell-bottoms
c) Bikini
d) Go-go boots

125. The 1960s saw the growth of a "flower power" movement, promoting what?
a) Technology
b) Military power
c) Peace and love
d) Industrial growth

126. Which British car, first launched in the 1960s, became an icon with its round headlights and compact design?
a) Volkswagen Beetle
b) Ford Mustang
c) Mini Cooper
d) Porsche 911

127. Which band sang about an "Aquarius" and the "dawning of the Age of Aquarius" in the 1960s?
a) The Mamas & the Papas
b) The 5th Dimension
c) Sonny & Cher
d) The Righteous Brothers

128. What did the "Peace Sign" symbolize in the 1960s?
a) Economic growth
b) Nuclear disarmament
c) Rapid urbanization
d) Industrialization

129. Which 1968 film featured the song "Raindrops Keep Fallin' on My Head"?
a) Midnight Cowboy
b) Butch Cassidy and the Sundance Kid
c) Easy Rider
d) Chitty Chitty Bang Bang

130. Who was the first American to orbit the Earth in 1962?
a) Neil Armstrong
b) Alan Shepard
c) Buzz Aldrin
d) John Glenn

131. Which legendary boxer, known for his catchphrase "Float like a butterfly, sting like a bee," rose to fame in the 1960s?
a) Joe Frazier
b) George Foreman
c) Muhammad Ali
d) Mike Tyson

132. Which 1960s T.V. show featured a magical genie and her astronaut master?
a) Gilligan's Island
b) Bewitched
c) The Twilight Zone
d) I Dream of Jeannie

133. Which 1960s pop artist is best known for songs like "It's My Party" and "You Don't Own Me"?
a) Aretha Franklin
b) Diana Ross
c) Leslie Gore
d) Janis Joplin

134. What iconic public festival was held in San Francisco's Golden Gate Park in 1967, attracting thousands?
a) Burning Man Festival
b) Monterey Pop Festival
c) Human Be-In
d) Earth Day Celebration

135. In which 1969 event did people gather to watch the launch of Apollo 11?
a) The Great American Eclipse
b) The Meteor Shower Festival
c) Moon Watch Party
d) Stars Gaze Night

136. Who hosted the 1960s TV show with puppet "Topo Gigio"?
a) Johnny Carson
b) Ed Sullivan
c) Dick Clark
d) Bob Barker

137. Which 1960s band had a hit with the song "California Dreamin'"?
a) The Byrds
b) The Mamas & the Papas
c) The Beach Boys
d) The Eagles

138. Who starred as the titular character in the 1960s television show "Bewitched"?
a) Lucille Ball
b) Elizabeth Montgomery
c) Donna Reed
d) Mary Tyler Moore

139. What was the primary goal of NASA's Apollo program in the 1960s?
a) Sending a probe to Mars
b) Building a space station
c) Landing a man on the Moon
d) Establishing a base on Venus

140. In 1968, which singer released the hit song "What a Wonderful World"?
a) Frank Sinatra
b) Bing Crosby
c) Louis Armstrong
d) Nat King Cole

141. What new dance was popularized by Chubby Checker in the early '60s?
a) The Macarena
b) The Twist
c) The Chicken Dance
d) The Salsa

142. Which colorful and psychedelic animated movie featuring The Beatles was released in 1968?
a) Help!
b) A Hard Day's Night
c) Let It Be
d) Yellow Submarine

143. What major event celebrated cultural and musical expression over three days in August 1969?
a) The Monterey Pop Festival
b) The Newport Folk Festival
c) Woodstock
d) The U.S. Festival

144. What was the name of the first James Bond film, released in 1962?
a) Goldfinger
b) Dr. No
c) From Russia With Love
d) Thunderball

145. In 1960, which athlete broke the four-minute mile record?
a) Steve Ovett
b) Roger Bannister
c) Sebastian Coe
d) Jim Ryun

146. Which iconic toy, introduced in the 1960s, allowed children to create glowing art using colored pegs?
a) Lite-Brite
b) Etch A Sketch
c) Spirograph
d) Magic Slate

147. What home-selling parties gained popularity in the 1960s?
a) Avon Parties
b) Tupperware Parties
c) Mary Kay Parties
d) Book Clubs

148. Which 1960s musical tells the story of a young woman arriving in New York with aspirations to be a nun?
a) The Sound of Music
b) Fiddler on the Roof
c) West Side Story
d) My Fair Lady

149. The 1960s "British Invasion" was a significant influence on which aspect of American culture?
a) Literature
b) Fashion
c) Politics
d) Music

150. Which 1960s cartoon series featured a family living in the Stone Age?
a) The Jetsons
b) The Flintstones
c) The Smurfs
d) ThunderCats

151. In 1964, what significant civil rights bill did President Lyndon B. Johnson enact into law?
a) Voting Rights Act
b) Civil Rights Act
c) Emancipation Proclamation
d) Equal Rights Amendment

152. Which 1960s fashion trend involved wearing pants that flared out from the knees down?
a) Hot pants
b) Go-go boots
c) Bell-bottoms
d) Mini-skirts

153. In the 1960s, what candy began using the slogan "Melts in your mouth, not in your hands"?
a) Skittles
b) M&Ms
c) Starburst
d) Reese's Pieces

154. Which 1960s T.V. show, set in space, featured characters named Captain Kirk and Spock?
a) Battlestar Galactica
b) The Twilight Zone
c) Star Wars
d) Star Trek

155. Which Disney theme park in Florida opened in 1965?
a) Epcot
b) Disney's Animal Kingdom
c) Disney's Hollywood Studios
d) Walt Disney World

156. The television show "Star Trek," premiering in the 60s, was set in which century?
a) 21st Century
b) 23rd Century
c) 25th Century
d) 20th Century

157. Which astronaut declared "That's one small step for man, one giant leap for mankind" in 1969?
a) Alan Shepard
b) Michael Collins
c) Buzz Aldrin
d) Neil Armstrong

158. Which Indian music instrument, like the sitar, gained popularity in the 1960s?
a) Kirtan
b) Raga
c) Bhajan
d) Ghazal

159. What 1967 San Francisco event celebrated music, art, and counterculture?
a) Haight Street Fair
b) Summer of Love
c) Woodstock
d) Monterey Pop Festival

160. Which '60s television show took viewers to a magical place where a twitching nose made things happen?
a) The Munsters
b) Bewitched
c) The Addams Family
d) I Dream of Jeannie

THE SUPER SEVENTIES

161. Which band released the hit album "Rumours" in 1977?
a) Fleetwood Mac
b) ABBA
c) The Eagles
d) Pink Floyd

162. Which 1971 film, starring Gene Wilder, is about a young boy's journey in a chocolate factory?
a) The Candy Man
b) Sweet Adventure
c) Chocolat
d) Willy Wonka & the Chocolate Factory

163. Which tennis player won the Wimbledon men's singles title in 1975?
a) Björn Borg
b) Jimmy Connors
c) Rod Laver
d) John McEnroe

164. Which car became an icon in the 1970s, known for its unique rotary engine?
a) Volkswagen Beetle
b) Ford Mustang
c) Mazda RX-7
d) Chevrolet Camaro

165. Which 70s game involves answering questions in the form of a question?
a) Wheel of Fortune
b) Jeopardy!
c) Family Feud
d) The Price Is Right

166. Which sitcom, premiering in 1971, featured a family named the Bradys?
a) Happy Days
b) The Partridge Family
c) The Brady Bunch
d) All in the Family

167. Which 1973 film is about a cop named "Popeye" Doyle?
a) The Sting
b) Bullitt
c) Serpico
d) The French Connection

168. What was the main setting for the 70s T.V. show "MAS*H"?
a) Police precinct
b) Army hospital
c) High school
d) Newsroom

169. Which soft-rock duo sang the 1970 hit "Close to You"?
a) Simon & Garfunkel
b) Sonny & Cher
c) The Carpenters
d) Captain & Tennille

170. In the 70s, people often sported shirts with what kind of wide, flaring collars?
a) Ascots
b) Band collars
c) Peter Pan collars
d) Butterfly collars

171. Which U.S. president declared July 20 as "Space Exploration Day" in honor of the Apollo 11 moon landing anniversary?
a) Gerald Ford
b) Richard Nixon
c) Jimmy Carter
d) Ronald Reagan

172. Which movie, released in 1975, made many people afraid to go into the water?
a) Jaws
b) The Deep
c) Orca
d) Piranha

173. **Which band sang the 1979 hit "Another Brick in the Wall"?**
a) Queen
b) The Who
c) Led Zeppelin
d) Pink Floyd

174. **Which 70s toy consisted of a spool that traveled up and down strings?**
a) Pet Rock
b) Rubik's Cube
c) Yo-Yo
d) Klackers

175. **The T.V. mini-series "Roots," aired in 1977, was based on a novel by which author?**
a) Toni Morrison
b) Alex Haley
c) James Baldwin
d) Maya Angelou

176. **In which 1978 movie did John Travolta and Olivia Newton-John star as high school sweethearts?**
a) Saturday Night Fever
b) Grease
c) Xanadu
d) Staying Alive

177. Which company introduced the first commercially available video game system, the Home Pong, in the 70s?
a) Nintendo
b) Sega
c) Atari
d) Magnavox

178. Which iconic 70s toy allowed children to create glowing art using colored pegs?
a) Spirograph
b) Etch A Sketch
c) Lite-Brite
d) Play-Doh Fun Factory

179. In the 1970s, which television series centered around a female detective agency overseen by the enigmatic Charlie?
a) Charlie's Angels
b) The Bionic Woman
c) Wonder Woman
d) Hart to Hart

180. Which 1970s T.V. show followed the lives of the Ingalls family in Walnut Grove?
a) The Waltons
b) Little House on the Prairie
c) Bonanza
d) The Ponderosa

181. The 1972 hit "American Pie" is a song by which artist?
a) Don McLean
b) Bob Dylan
c) Jim Croce
d) Neil Diamond

182. Which disco sensation performed the 1978 hit "I Will Survive"?
a) Gloria Gaynor
b) Diana Ross
c) Donna Summer
d) Chaka Khan

183. The 1970s dance known as "The Bump" involved what kind of movement?
a) Handclaps
b) Foot stomping
c) Hip thrusts
d) Head nods

184. Which 1970s film follows a young woman named Fanny Brice and her rise to fame?
a) Cabaret
b) A Star is Born
c) Funny Girl
d) My Fair Lady

185. Which celebrity was known for his signature jump-suits and capes during the 1970s?
a) Elton John
b) Freddie Mercury
c) Elvis Presley
d) Mick Jagger

186. The 1977 Mini-Series "Roots" traced the history of which family over several generations?
a) Kinte
b) Jefferson
c) Williams
d) Turner

187. Which iconic character, first appearing in the 1970s, was known for his catchphrase "Hey, hey, hey!"?
a) Fred Flintstone
b) Fat Albert
c) Scooby-Doo
d) Kermit the Frog

188. Which 1970s sci-fi movie was taglined "A long time ago in a galaxy far, far away..."?
a) Star Trek
b) Flash Gordon
c) Close Encounters of the Third Kind
d) Star Wars

189. Which American swimmer won seven gold medals at the 1972 Munich Olympics?
a) Greg Louganis
b) Ian Thorpe
c) Mark Spitz
d) Michael Phelps

190. The Ford Pinto, a popular compact car, was introduced in which year of the 1970s?
a) 1970
b) 1974
c) 1976
d) 1978

191. Which 1970s T.V. show was set on the S.S. Minnow, a shipwrecked boat?
a) Fantasy Island
b) The Love Boat
c) Gilligan's Island
d) The S.S. Adventure

192. Who sang the 1973 hit "Killing Me Softly with His Song"?
a) Carly Simon
b) Joni Mitchell
c) Roberta Flack
d) Karen Carpenter

193. Which 1970s children's show featured a big yellow bird and a grouch who lived in a trash can?
a) Mister Rogers' Neighborhood
b) The Muppet Show
c) Sesame Street
d) Captain Kangaroo

194. Who starred as the titular character in the 1976 film "Rocky"?
a) Al Pacino
b) Robert De Niro
c) Sylvester Stallone
d) Burt Reynolds

195. In the 70s, many people sported a type of jeans that flared out from the knees. What were they called?
a) Bell-bottoms
b) Jeggings
c) Boot cut
d) High-rise

196. The 1976 Summer Olympics were held in which city?
a) Moscow
b) Los Angeles
c) Munich
d) Montreal

197. Which popular 70s dance was characterized by a "hustle step"?
a) The Bop
b) The Twist
c) The Macarena
d) The Hustle

198. Which T.V. show followed the paranormal investigations of two agents named Mulder and Scully?
a) The Twilight Zone
b) The X-Files
c) Outer Limits
d) Twin Peaks

199. Which 70s movie has a famous bicycle flying scene across the moon?
a) Close Encounters of the Third Kind
b) Star Wars
c) E.T. the Extra-Terrestrial
d) Alien

200. In which sport did Björn Borg make significant waves during the 70s?
a) Golf
b) Tennis
c) Boxing
d) Swimming

201. The A.M.C. Gremlin, a distinctive looking compact car, was introduced in which year of the 1970s?
a) 1970
b) 1972
c) 1975
d) 1978

202. Which 1970s variety show featured a country singer and her family, including a segment titled "Pickin' and Grinnin'"?
a) The Cher Show
b) The Johnny Cash Show
c) Hee Haw
d) The Dolly Parton Show

203. Which company introduced the first personal computer in 1977?
a) I.B.M.
b) Microsoft
c) Apple
d) Commodore

204. Which 1970s animated series featured a futuristic family living in Orbit City?
a) Thunderbirds
b) The Flintstones
c) The Jetsons
d) Transformers

205. Who became the World Chess Champion in 1972, defeating Boris Spassky?
a) Garry Kasparov
b) Anatoly Karpov
c) Magnus Carlsen
d) Bobby Fischer

206. The 1970s "Pet Rock" fad offered a pet that was what?
a) Easy to care for
b) Actually a rock
c) Colorful
d) Soft and cuddly

207. Which American band released the 1976 album "Hotel California"?
a) The Doors
b) The Eagles
c) The Beach Boys
d) Grateful Dead

208. Which 1970s T.V. show featured an alien named Mork?
a) Alf
b) Third Rock from the Sun
c) Mork & Mindy
d) My Favorite Martian

209. The 1970s saw the rise of a new home video format. What was it called?
a) DVD
b) Laserdisc
c) VHS
d) Blu-ray

210. Which of these artists painted the famous 1971 work "The Persistence of Plastic"?
a) Roy Lichtenstein
b) Andy Warhol
c) Pablo Picasso
d) Jackson Pollock

211. The 1970s popular toy Lite-Brite allowed kids to create pictures using what?
a) Magnetic pieces
b) Colored water
c) Illuminated pegs
d) Etching lines

212. Which iconic 70s movie is known for the quote, "You talkin' to me?"?
a) The Godfather
b) Jaws
c) Taxi Driver
d) A Clockwork Orange

213. Which magazine, first published in the 1970s, was aimed at providing tech enthusiasts with D.I.Y. electronics projects?
a) Wired
b) Byte
c) Popular Mechanics
d) MAKE

214. Which 1970s disco club in New York became famous for its celebrity guests and Studio 54 dancers?
a) The Roxy
b) CBGB
c) The Limelight
d) Studio 54

215. Who won the Best Actress Oscar in 1977 for her role in "Network"?
a) Sally Field
b) Diane Keaton
c) Faye Dunaway
d) Jane Fonda

216. Which 1970s children's toy featured a face made of vegetables and fruits on a spud?
a) Cabbage Patch Kids
b) Mr. Potato Head
c) Care Bears
d) Strawberry Shortcake

217. Which 1970s fashion trend involved trousers that became wider from the knees downward?
a) Pegged pants
b) Bell-bottoms
c) Capris
d) Culottes

218. Which 1970s toy allowed players to mold shapes using heated plastic goop?
a) Easy-Bake Oven
b) Spirograph
c) ThingMaker
d) Silly Putty

219. Which music genre gained massive popularity in the 70s, featuring artists like Gloria Gaynor and the Bee Gees?
a) Punk rock
b) Disco
c) Grunge
d) New wave

220. Which 1970s T.V. show was set in a cab company called the Sunshine Cab Company?
a) Cheers
b) Taxi
c) WKRP in Cincinnati
d) Night Court

221. Which hairstyle, popular in the 70s, featured hair tightly curled into small, dense ringlets?
a) Perm
b) Mullet
c) Afro
d) Shag

222. In which 1970s board game do players acquire property and aim to bankrupt opponents?
a) Clue
b) Monopoly
c) Scrabble
d) Life

223. The Pontiac Firebird is associated with which iconic 1970s movie featuring Burt Reynolds?
a) Bullitt
b) The French Connection
c) Smokey and the Bandit
d) Cannonball Run

224. Which artist is famous for his 1970s hits "Maggie May" and "Tonight's the Night"?
a) Rod Stewart
b) Elton John
c) David Bowie
d) Bruce Springsteen

225. Which music festival, held in 1970, is often referred to as "the U.K.'s Woodstock"?
a) Glastonbury
b) Reading
c) Isle of Wight
d) Lollapalooza

226. Which 1970s sitcom chronicled the misadventures of two single women and their neighbors in Minneapolis?
a) Golden Girls
b) Mary Tyler Moore Show
c) Laverne & Shirley
d) The Carol Burnett Show

227. Which iconic 70s soda was promoted as "The Uncola"?
a) Dr. Pepper
b) Pepsi
c) 7-Up
d) Coca-Cola

228. The 1970s Pulsar watch was revolutionary because it was the first to display what?
a) Moon phases
b) Digital numbers
c) Dual time zones
d) Atomic time synchronization

229. Which 1970s T.V. detective was known for his rumpled raincoat and cigar?
a) Kojak
b) Magnum, P.I.
c) Columbo
d) Rockford

230. Which 1970s toy promised "A race for fun, but watch your thumb!"?
a) Simon
b) Bop It
c) Hungry Hungry Hippos
d) Whac-A-Mole

231. Which 70s musical group featured three brothers with the last name Gibb?
a) The Osmonds
b) Bee Gees
c) The Jackson 5
d) The Doobie Brothers

232. The Polaroid SX-70, introduced in the 1970s, was a revolutionary type of what?
a) Television
b) Radio
c) Camera
d) Phonograph

233. Which band released the hit song "Stayin' Alive" in the late 70s?
a) The Rolling Stones
b) Bee Gees
c) ABBA
d) Queen

234. Which T.V. show debuted in the 70s and took place on a cruise ship?
a) The Love Boat
b) Fantasy Island
c) Baywatch
d) Voyage to the Bottom of the Sea

235. In which movie does the character Tony Manero showcase his disco dancing skills?
a) Saturday Night Fever
b) Grease
c) Flashdance
d) Footloose

236. Which tennis player won the Wimbledon Women's Singles title nine times, beginning in the 70s?
a) Maria Bueno
b) Billie Jean King
c) Martina Navratilova
d) Chris Evert

237. Which American city was known as the birthplace of the disco movement in the 70s?
a) Chicago
b) Los Angeles
c) New York City
d) Miami

238. Which car was the best-selling model in the United States during the 70s?
a) Chevrolet Impala
b) Ford Pinto
c) Volkswagen Beetle
d) Toyota Corolla

239. Which 1970s fashion item was characterized by its bell shape at the bottom?
a) Bell-bottom pants
b) Ponchos
c) Tube tops
d) Platform shoes

240. What was the popular 70s dance that involved pointing a finger up and down?
a) Moonwalk
b) Robot
c) YMCA
d) Running Man

THE ELECTRIC EIGHTIES

241. Which 1980s T.V. show featured a talking car named KITT?

a) Miami Vice
b) Knight Rider
c) Magnum, P.I.
d) Airwolf

242. Who sang the 1980s hit song "Material Girl"?
a) Cyndi Lauper
b) Whitney Houston
c) Madonna
d) Tina Turner

243. Which game console was released by Nintendo in the 1980s, becoming an instant hit?
a) Atari 2600
b) Sega Genesis
c) N.E.S. (Nintendo Entertainment System)
d) PlayStation

244. In which 80s movie did a young Tom Cruise dance in his living room in just a shirt and socks?
a) Top Gun
b) Rain Man
c) Risky Business
d) Cocktail

245. Which aerobic workout became popular in the 1980s thanks to videos and T.V. shows?
a) Zumba
b) CrossFit
c) Jazzercise
d) Pilates

246. Who starred as the title character in the 1980s sitcom "A.L.F.", about an alien living with a suburban family?
a) Max Wright
b) Paul Fusco
c) Michael J. Fox
d) Tony Danza

247. Which 80s movie featured the characters Marty McFly and Doc Brown traveling through time?
a) Ghostbusters
b) The Breakfast Club
c) Blade Runner
d) Back to the Future

248. Which toy cube puzzle became a worldwide craze in the 1980s?
a) Bop It
b) Rubik's Cube
c) Simon
d) Tamagotchi

249. Which of these bands did NOT hail from the U.K. during the 1980s music scene?
a) Duran Duran
b) Depeche Mode
c) R.E.M.
d) The Cure

250. Which fashion accessory became popular in the 80s and was often brightly colored and made of rubber?
a) Jelly sandals
b) Scrunchies
c) Leg warmers
d) Shoulder pads

251. Which famous artist painted the Campbell's Soup Cans and became an icon of the 1980s art scene?
a) Salvador Dalí
b) Pablo Picasso
c) Roy Lichtenstein
d) Andy Warhol

252. Which 1980s video game features a yellow character that eats dots and avoids ghosts?
a) Tetris
b) Super Mario Bros.
c) Pac-Man
d) Space Invaders

253. Which T.V. family from the 80s lived in a home located in San Francisco?
a) The Huxtables ("The Cosby Show")
b) The Keatons ("Family Ties")
c) The Tanners ("Full House")
d) The Seavers ("Growing Pains")

254. Which aerobic workout became wildly popular in the 80s, led by an energetic man in striped shorts?
a) Billy's Bootcamp
b) The Richard Simmons Show
c) Jane Fonda's Workout
d) Buns of Steel

255. Which T.V. show, set in a bar in Boston, had the tagline, "Where everybody knows your name"?
a) MAS*H
b) Cheers
c) The Golden Girls
d) The A-Team

256. Which 80s toy was known for its tagline, "Transformers, robots in disguise"?
a) He-Man
b) G.I. Joe
c) Voltron
d) Transformers

257. Which 1980s film features five high school students serving detention on a Saturday?
a) Sixteen Candles
b) Ferris Bueller's Day Off
c) Fast Times at Ridgemont High
d) The Breakfast Club

258. Whose 1984 hit single was titled "What's Love Got to Do with It"?
a) Madonna
b) Cyndi Lauper
c) Tina Turner
d) Whitney Houston

259. Which iconic '80s arcade game tasks players with guiding a frog safely across a bustling street?
a) Q*bert
b) Donkey Kong
c) Frogger
d) Space Invaders

260. Which hairstyle, popular in the 80s, involves shaving one side of the head?
a) Mohawk
b) Rat tail
c) Mullet
d) Skrillex

261. Which 80s T.V. show starred Michael J. Fox as Alex P. Keaton?
a) Who's the Boss?
b) Family Ties
c) Alf
d) Silver Spoons

262. Which cartoon featured feline characters from the planet Thundera?
a) He-Man
b) Voltron
c) ThunderCats
d) Transformers

263. Which 'Walkman' company revolutionized personal audio in the 1980s?
a) Philips
b) Toshiba
c) Sony
d) Panasonic

264. Which car became famous in the 80s for its gull-wing doors and its role in a popular film series?
a) Chevrolet Camaro
b) Pontiac Firebird
c) Ford Mustang
d) DeLorean DMC-12

265. What was the name of the dance that became a craze after a song by Los del Río was released in the 80s?
a) Cha-Cha Slide
b) Electric Slide
c) Macarena
d) The Hustle

266. Which '80s movie is centered around a dance ban in a small town?
a) Flashdance
b) Dirty Dancing
c) Footloose
d) Saturday Night Fever

267. Which 80s toy allowed kids to mold shapes using colored plastic goop and a heated mold?
a) Creepy Crawlers
b) Lite Brite
c) Silly Putty
d) Play-Doh Fun Factory

268. Which artist's 1984 album "Purple Rain" became a massive hit?
a) Michael Jackson
b) Prince
c) Bruce Springsteen
d) David Bowie

269. Which game, introduced in the '80s, involved catching a variety of creatures with colorful, spring-loaded traps?
a) Mouse Trap
b) Hungry Hungry Hippos
c) Connect Four
d) Operation

270. Which music channel was launched in 1981, revolutionizing the music and television industries?
a) VH1
b) B.E.T.
c) MTV
d) CMT

271. Which fitness guru launched a series of aerobics videos in the 1980s?
a) Jillian Michaels
b) Billy Blanks
c) Richard Simmons
d) Jane Fonda

272. In the 1980s, what was the primary purpose of a 'Swatch'?
a) To make phone calls
b) To tell time
c) To play music
d) To take photos

273. Which popular 80s toy had a catchy jingle that claimed they were "so soft, cuddly, and cute"?
a) Teddy Ruxpin
b) Pound Puppies
c) My Little Pony
d) Cabbage Patch Kids

274. In which '80s film does a young boy befriend an alien and try to help him return home?
a) Close Encounters of the Third Kind
b) E.T. the Extra-Terrestrial
c) The Thing
d) Starman

275. Which of these actors did NOT star in the Brat Pack movies of the 1980s?
a) Emilio Estevez
b) Rob Lowe
c) Matthew Broderick
d) Molly Ringwald

276. Which soda introduced the "Choice of a New Generation" campaign in the 1980s?
a) Coca-Cola
b) Dr. Pepper
c) Pepsi
d) Sprite

277. What was the handheld electronic game in the 80s where players could "travel" Oregon Trail?
a) Game Boy
b) Atari Lynx
c) TurboExpress
d) MECC

278. Which fashion accessory became popular in the 80s and was often brightly colored or patterned?
a) Bell bottoms
b) Leg warmers
c) Bow ties
d) Poodle skirts

279. Which band had a huge hit in the 80s with "Every Breath You Take"?
a) U2
b) The Rolling Stones
c) The Police
d) Duran Duran

280. What was the name of the 1980s personal computer introduced by Apple?
a) Apple Core
b) Apple I
c) Macintosh
d) Apple IIe

281. Which 80s T.V. series followed the lives of the Ewing family in Texas?
a) Dynasty
b) Dallas
c) Falcon Crest
d) Knots Landing

282. Which cartoon featured a group of heroes who said, "By the power of Grayskull!"?
a) ThunderCats
b) G.I. Joe
c) He-Man and the Masters of the Universe
d) Transformers

283. Who hosted the 1980s children's program "Reading Rainbow"?
a) Bill Nye
b) Fred Rogers
c) LeVar Burton
d) Bob Ross

284. Which 80s toy let children create pictures by poking small, colored pegs into a board?
a) Spirograph
b) Etch A Sketch
c) Lite-Brite
d) Rubik's Cube

285. Which iconic 80s song begins with the line "Just a small town girl, living in a lonely world"?
a) "Girls Just Want to Have Fun"
b) "Sweet Child o' Mine"
c) "Don't Stop Believing"
d) "Like a Virgin"

286. What item did Marty McFly famously ride on in "Back to the Future"?
a) A scooter
b) A skateboard
c) A bicycle
d) A rollerblade

287. Which 1980s toy could be "cuddled and fed" and came with an adoption certificate?
a) Furby
b) Cabbage Patch Kids
c) Care Bears
d) Trolls

288. Which 80s band is known for hits like "Rio" and "Hungry Like the Wolf"?
a) A-ha
b) Wham!
c) Duran Duran
d) Culture Club

289. Which 80s arcade game had players defending earth from aliens?
a) Pong
b) Centipede
c) Galaga
d) Tetris

290. Which 80s T.V. show was set on a remote Hawaiian estate and followed the adventures of a private investigator?
a) Miami Vice
b) Hawaii Five-O
c) Magnum P.I.
d) Simon & Simon

291. Which 80s soft drink, labeled "New," was swiftly replaced after public backlash?
a) Pepsi Clear
b) Coca-Cola Classic
c) New Coke
d) Dr. Pepper Gold

292. In which film from the 1980s do children embark on a quest for pirate gold to prevent the loss of their homes?
a) Stand By Me
b) The Lost Boys
c) The Goonies
d) Explorers

293. In which video 80s game does a character save a princess from a giant gorilla?
a) Super Mario Bros.
b) Donkey Kong
c) Zelda
d) Mega Man

294. What was the name of Michael Jackson's 1982 album, which became one of the best-selling albums of all time?
a) "Thriller"
b) "Bad"
c) "Off the Wall"
d) "Dangerous"

295. Which toy, popularized in the 80s, consisted of a bouncy ball with a handle that children could sit on and hop around with?
a) Pogo Ball
b) Space Hopper
c) Skip-It
d) Bop It

296. Which 1980s sitcom was set in a Boston bar "where everybody knows your name"?
a) MAS*H
b) Cheers
c) Full House
d) The Golden Girls

297. What handheld electronic game, introduced in the 80s, challenged players to repeat a sequence of colored lights and sounds?
a) Simon
b) Tamagotchi
c) Game Boy
d) Speak & Spell

298. Which artist sang the 80s hit "Like a Prayer"?
a) Whitney Houston
b) Cyndi Lauper
c) Madonna
d) Cher

299. Which T.V. alien often used the phrase "Nanu Nanu"?
a) A.L.F.
b) Mork
c) Spock
d) Gizmo

300. The Sony Walkman, introduced in the 80s, allowed people to:
a) Make phone calls
b) Play video games
c) Listen to music on the go
d) Take photographs

301. Which toy robot was known for its catchphrase "It's fun to play with, not to eat!"?
a) Teddy Ruxpin
b) Transformers
c) My Buddy
d) Mr. Potato Head

302. What 1980s aerobics workout grew popular through a series of videotapes?
a) Jazzercise
b) Tae Bo
c) Zumba
d) Pilates

303. Which '80s fantasy film features a young Jennifer Connelly navigating a labyrinth to rescue her baby brother?
a) The Princess Bride
b) Labyrinth
c) Willow
d) The Dark Crystal

304. What's the title of the 1984 song that encouraged listeners to "take on me"?
a) Jump
b) Wake Me Up Before You Go-Go
c) Take On Me
d) Sweet Dreams

305. In which 80s T.V. show did David Hasselhoff guard the beaches of Los Angeles?
a) Baywatch
b) Miami Vice
c) Hill Street Blues
d) Dynasty

306. What board game, popular in the 80s, involved hunting for treasure on an island as it sank?
a) Life
b) Forbidden Island
c) Treasure Hunt
d) Fireball Island

307. Which daytime drama set in a hospital premiered in the late 60s and gained immense popularity in the 80s?
a) The Bold and the Beautiful
b) Days of Our Lives
c) General Hospital
d) The Young and the Restless

308. What colorful 80s toy allowed kids to mold and bake their own designs?
a) Lite-Brite
b) Play-Doh
c) Silly Putty
d) Shrinky Dinks

309. Which 80s T.V. show featured a group of women working at a design firm in Atlanta?
a) Designing Women
b) Murphy Brown
c) The Facts of Life
d) Cagney & Lacey

310. What brand popularized high-top sneakers in the 1980s?
a) Reebok
b) Adidas
c) Nike
d) Converse

311. In the 80s, many kids played with these stackable, interlocking bricks. What are they called?
a) Lego
b) K'NEX
c) Tinkertoys
d) Lincoln Logs

312. Which 1980s T.V. family lived in San Francisco with their three daughters and Uncle Jesse?
a) The Seavers
b) The Tanners
c) The Keatons
d) The Huxtables

313. Which animated T.V. series in the 80s featured four amphibious warriors named after famous artists?
a) ThunderCats
b) He-Man and the Masters of the Universe
c) Teenage Mutant Ninja Turtles
d) The Transformers

314. Which toy became a sensation and involved "caring" for a furry creature that came with an adoption certificate?
a) Cabbage Patch Kids
b) My Little Pony
c) Pound Puppies
d) Care Bears

315. Which 80s game show had contestants "shop" in a fake store for prizes?
a) The Price Is Right
b) Wheel of Fortune
c) Supermarket Sweep
d) Let's Make a Deal

316. Who sang the iconic 1980's hit "Sweet Child o' Mine"?
a) Aerosmith
b) AC/DC
c) Guns N' Roses
d) Bon Jovi

317. In which 80s show did Alex P. Keaton often clash with his ex-hippie parents over his conservative views?
a) Who's the Boss?
b) Family Matters
c) Growing Pains
d) Family Ties

318. Which 80s dance craze featured side-to-side movements and hopping?
a) Electric Slide
b) Cabbage Patch
c) Moonwalk
d) Hammer Dance

319. What 80s T.V. show took place on the tropical estate of Robin Masters and featured a mustached detective?
a) Magnum, P.I.
b) Knight Rider
c) The A-Team
d) Miami Vice

320. Which 1980's dance move involved mimicking the motion of a robot?
a) Moonwalk
b) Breakdancing
c) Robot Dance
d) Worm

THE GREAT NINETIES

321. Which '90s T.V. show featured six friends living in New York and often meeting at a coffee shop called Central Perk?

a) Seinfeld
b) Cheers
c) Friends
d) Frasier

322. Which handheld digital pet was a huge hit in the 1990s?
a) Giga Pet
b) Furby
c) Neopet
d) Tamagotchi

323. In the '90s, which toy answered user questions with responses like "It is certain" or "Reply hazy, try again"?
a) Bop It
b) Magic 8-Ball
c) Simon
d) Rubik's Cube

324. Which song by Los Del Rio became a dance craze in the mid-'90s?
a) La Bamba
b) Despacito
c) Macarena
d) Bailando

325. What was the name of the purple dinosaur that taught children life lessons through songs?
a) Godzilla
b) Yoshi
c) Barney
d) Dino

326. Which shoe brand featured a thick sole and was worn by members of the Spice Girls?
a) Nike
b) Crocs
c) Dr. Martens
d) Platform shoes

327. Who was known as the "Fresh Prince" in a '90s sitcom?
a) Will Smith
b) Jazzy Jeff
c) Chris Rock
d) L.L. Cool J

328. Which '90s cartoon followed the lives of babies named Tommy, Chuckie, Phil, and Lil?
a) Doug
b) Hey Arnold!
c) Rugrats
d) Rocko's Modern Life

329. Which animated feature, released in 1994, told the story of a lion named Simba?
a) The Jungle Book
b) The Lion King
c) Madagascar
d) Tarzan

330. Which '90s band sang hits like "I Want it That Way" and "As Long as You Love Me"?
a) Backstreet Boys
b) NSYNC
c) New Kids on the Block
d) 98 Degrees

331. What game system was released by Sony in the mid-'90s, marking their entry into the console market?
a) Sega Genesis
b) Xbox
c) PlayStation
d) Nintendo 64

332. Which character was NOT a part of the popular '90s T.V. show "Power Rangers"?
a) Red Ranger
b) Pink Ranger
c) Aqua Ranger
d) Yellow Ranger

333. What toy featured a slippery, gel-filled rubber ball that was hard to grip?
a) Pogs
b) Slinky
c) Beanie Babies
d) Water Snake

334. What was the name of the toy that allowed children to draw with a spinning disk and colorful pens?
a) Sketch-a-Graph
b) Spirograph
c) Etch A Sketch
d) Spin Art

335. In the 1999 film "Toy Story 2," which new character, a cowgirl, was introduced?
a) Daisy
b) Bullseye
c) Bo Peep
d) Jessie

336. Which '90s T.V. game show required contestants to complete physical and mental challenges within a time limit inside a house?
a) The Crystal Maze
b) Double Dare
c) Legends of the Hidden Temple
d) Nickelodeon Guts

337. Which '90s computer game involved aligning falling blocks to complete rows?
a) Tetris
b) Minesweeper
c) Solitaire
d) Pong

338. What item, introduced in the '90s, could store a playlist of songs and skip without scratching?
a) Cassette player
b) Vinyl record
c) MP3 player
d) Compact Disc (CD) player

339. Which '90s sitcom took place in a fictional Boston bar where "everybody knows your name"?
a) Cheers
b) Frasier
c) The Drew Carey Show
d) Mork & Mindy

340. Which toy, popular in the '90s, featured small stuffed animals filled with "beans"?
a) Teddy Ruxpin
b) Cabbage Patch Kids
c) Furby
d) Beanie Babies

341. Which '90s T.V. show featured a teenage witch named Sabrina?
a) Buffy the Vampire Slayer
b) Charmed
c) Sabrina the Teenage Witch
d) The Craft

342. Which of these was NOT a flavor of the '90s drink Fruitopia?
a) Strawberry Passion Awareness
b) Grape Beyond
c) Tropical Fruit Fever
d) Mango Madness

343. Which basketball player starred alongside Bugs Bunny in the 1996 movie "Space Jam"?
a) Michael Jordan
b) Scottie Pippen
c) Kobe Bryant
d) Shaquille O'Neal

344. The '90s dance "The Macarena" originated in which country?
a) Italy
b) Brazil
c) Spain
d) Mexico

345. In 1991, which company introduced the world's first commercially available digital camera?
a) Canon
b) Nikon
c) Kodak
d) Sony

346. The hit song "MMMBop" was performed by which band of brothers?
a) Hanson
b) The Jonas Brothers
c) The Moffatts
d) The Jackson 5

347. Which animated T.V. show featured siblings named Phil and Lil?
a) Doug
b) Recess
c) The Powerpuff Girls
d) Rugrats

348. Which board game, released in the 90s, required players to guess their opponent's character based on appearance?
a) Guess Who?
b) Connect Four
c) Candy Land
d) Battleship

349. Who was the lead actor in the 1993 film "Jurassic Park"?
a) Jeff Goldblum
b) Harrison Ford
c) Tom Hanks
d) Sam Neill

350. What '90s toy was a colorful bear that glowed from a light inside its body?
a) Glow Worm
b) Teddy Ruxpin
c) Care Bear
d) Tickle Me Elmo

351. In which '90s film did Robin Williams play a grown-up Peter Pan returning to Neverland?
a) Hook
b) Jumanji
c) Mrs. Doubtfire
d) Dead Poets Society

352. Which character is known for his catchphrase "Did I do that?" in a '90s sitcom?
a) Joey Tribbiani
b) Urkel
c) Tim "The Toolman" Taylor
d) Chandler Bing

353. Which T.V. show featured a group of teens with the ability to "morph" into different animals to fight off alien invaders?
a) Animorphs
b) Goosebumps
c) Are You Afraid of the Dark?
d) ThunderCats

354. Which band released the hit song "Wonderwall" in the '90s?
a) Blur
b) The Verve
c) Oasis
d) Radiohead

355. Which of these is NOT a '90s Beanie Baby?
a) Princess the Bear
b) Patti the Platypus
c) Legs the Frog
d) Larry the Llama

356. Which '90s video game console had a mascot named Sonic?
a) Nintendo 64
b) PlayStation
c) Atari Jaguar
d) Sega Genesis

357. What '90s toy required careful balance to keep its two foot platforms level while stepping?
a) Bop It
b) Skip-It
c) Pogo Ball
d) Moon Shoes

358. In the '90s, which cereal introduced a mascot named "Chip the Wolf"?
a) Lucky Charms
b) Cookie Crisp
c) Golden Grahams
d) Cinnamon Toast Crunch

359. Which '90s T.V. show was set at Bayside High School?
a) Boy Meets World
b) Saved by the Bell
c) Fresh Prince of Bel-Air
d) 90210

360. What popular '90s toy was a squishy, stretchy action figure filled with gel?
a) Beanie Babies
b) Silly Putty
c) Polly Pocket
d) Stretch Armstrong

361. Which hit song features the lyrics, "It's a beautiful life, oh oh oh oh"?
a) "Blue (Da Ba Dee)" - Eiffel 65
b) "Barbie Girl" - Aqua
c) "Beautiful Life" - Ace of Base
d) "What is Love" – Haddaway

362. The '90s fashion trend "JNCO Jeans" was known for what distinct feature?
a) Extremely wide legs
b) High waists
c) Acid wash finish
d) Built-in suspenders

363. Which show featured a coffee shop called "Central Perk"?
a) The X-Files
b) Friends
c) Frasier
d) Will & Grace

364. The 1992 Summer Olympics, where professional basketball players from the N.B.A. participated for the first time, was held in which city?
a) Atlanta
b) Sydney
c) Barcelona
d) Seoul

365. Who sang the theme song for "The Fresh Prince of Bel-Air"?
a) Will Smith
b) L.L. Cool J
c) D.J. Jazzy Jeff
d) MC Hammer

366. Which toy featured colorful interlocking plastic bricks and was popularized in the '90s, though it was invented much earlier?
a) Lincoln Logs
b) Playmobil
c) LEGO
d) K'NEX

367. In the 1990 movie "Pretty Woman," who played the lead role of Vivian Ward?
a) Meg Ryan
b) Julia Roberts
c) Sandra Bullock
d) Nicole Kidman

368. Which '90s band is known for their hit "Don't Speak"?
a) No Doubt
b) Spice Girls
c) Backstreet Boys
d) Destiny's Child

369. In 1998, which search engine company was founded by Larry Page and Sergey Brin?
a) Yahoo
b) Bing
c) Google
d) Ask Jeeves

370. Which soda was introduced in the '90s as a clear alternative to colas?
a) Sprite
b) Pepsi Blue
c) 7-Up
d) Crystal Pepsi

371. Which children's book series, written by R.L. Stine, spooked readers throughout the '90s?
a) The Babysitters Club
b) Nancy Drew
c) Goosebumps
d) Hardy Boys

372. What handheld digital pet, which you had to feed and clean up after, was launched in the '90s?
a) Aibo
b) Furbies
c) Giga Pets
d) Neopets

373. Which of these Disney movies was NOT released in the 1990s?
a) The Lion King
b) Beauty and the Beast
c) The Little Mermaid
d) Mulan

374. Who was known as the "Queen of Pop" in the '90s?
a) Whitney Houston
b) Mariah Carey
c) Madonna
d) Celine Dion

375. What was the name of the butler in the T.V. show "The Nanny"?
a) Geoffrey
b) Winston
c) Niles
d) Alfred

376. In the '90s, which company used the slogan "Think Different"?
a) I.B.M.
b) Microsoft
c) Apple
d) Google

377. Which '90s T.V. show starred Sarah Michelle Gellar as a vampire slayer?
a) Charmed
b) Angel
c) Buffy the Vampire Slayer
d) Roswell

378. Which band had a hit in the '90s with the song "Wannabe"?
a) T.L.C.
b) Destiny's Child
c) Spice Girls
d) Salt-N-Pepa

379. The Tamagotchi, a virtual pet, originated from which country in the '90s?
a) South Korea
b) China
c) Japan
d) United States

380. In which '90s movie did Tom Hanks play a character stranded on an island?
a) Cast Away
b) Forrest Gump
c) Philadelphia
d) Sleepless in Seattle

381. What was the name of the popular '90s toy that responded to voice commands and could "learn" over time?
a) Tickle Me Elmo
b) Furbies
c) Beanie Babies
d) Tamagotchi

382. The '90s video game console, PlayStation, was released by which company?
a) Nintendo
b) Sega
c) Microsoft
d) Sony

383. Which of the following movies did NOT star Julia Roberts in the '90s?
a) Notting Hill
b) Erin Brockovich
c) Runaway Bride
d) The Proposal

384. The 'Macarena' dance craze was popularized by which artist(s)?
a) Ricky Martin
b) Gloria Estefan
c) Los Del Rio
d) Enrique Iglesias

385. Which of the following was a popular '90s chat program?
a) Skype
b) WhatsApp
c) AOL Instant Messenger (A.I.M.)
d) Snapchat

386. In 1997, which British author released the first book in a series about a young wizard?
a) J.R.R. Tolkien
b) J.K. Rowling
c) Suzanne Collins
d) Philip Pullman

387. Which athlete, nicknamed "Air", was renowned for his basketball skills in the '90s?
a) LeBron James
b) Magic Johnson
c) Kobe Bryant
d) Michael Jordan

388. The T.V. show "Baywatch" prominently featured which beach?
a) Miami Beach
b) Malibu Beach
c) Bondi Beach
d) Myrtle Beach

389. Which '90s animated film featured a soundtrack hit, "Circle of Life"?
a) The Little Mermaid
b) The Lion King
c) Aladdin
d) Pocahontas

390. Which '90s toy allowed kids to create 3D plastic designs using templates and a special oven?
a) Spirograph
b) Creepy Crawlers
c) Lite Brite
d) Shrinky Dinks

391. Which '90s toy featured a small piece of cardboard that you could "slap" onto your wrist, and it would wrap around it?
a) Slap Bracelets
b) Pogs
c) Loom Bands
d) Magic Grow Capsules

392. The '90s saw the rise of which digital assistant, known for its paperclip avatar?
a) Google Assistant
b) Siri
c) Alexa
d) Clippy

393. What '90s T.V. show featured a talking baby named Maggie, who often tried to escape her playpen?
a) Family Guy
b) The Simpsons
c) South Park
d) Rugrats

394. In the late '90s, which company introduced the iMac, a personal computer with a distinctive transparent colored design?
a) Microsoft
b) Dell
c) Apple
d) IBM

395. In 1991, which artist released the album "Diamonds and Pearls"?
a) Michael Jackson
b) Prince
c) Madonna
d) George Michael

396. Which '90s T.V. show focused on FBI agents investigating unexplained phenomena?
a) X-Files
b) Unsolved Mysteries
c) Twilight Zone
d) Outer Limits

397. Who was known as the "Fresh Prince" in a '90s T.V. show?
a) Will Smith
b) Jazzy Jeff
c) Eddie Murphy
d) Martin Lawrence

398. Which '90s Disney movie features the character named Quasimodo?
a) Pocahontas
b) Beauty and the Beast
c) The Little Mermaid
d) The Hunchback of Notre Dame

399. Which '90s sitcom was centered around the lives of the employees of a fictional news radio station?
a) Just Shoot Me!
b) NewsRadio
c) The Larry Sanders Show
d) Frasier

400. Which '90s movie is about a young girl who discovers a board game that comes to life?
a) The Game
b) The Matrix
c) Clue
d) Jumanji

SHARE YOUR THOUGHTS!

Dear Reader,

Have you finished the book? We'd love to hear your take on it! Please consider leaving an honest review because your feedback guides other readers and helps us grow.

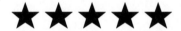

How to Leave a Review

Scan the QR code, which will take you to the review page.

Your voice matters. Lend it to the conversation and help shape future reads!

Thank you.

ANSWERS

1. c) Hula hoop
2. c) Dwight D. Eisenhower
3. b) A Streetcar Named Desire
4. c) Elvis Presley
5. c) Ran a mile in under four minutes
6. d) I Love Lucy
7. b) Climb Mount Everest
8. c) Disneyland
9. c) Chevrolet Corvette
10. d) The Catcher in the Rye
11. c) James Dean
12. b) I Love Lucy
13. a) The Twist (popularized in the early 1960s)
14. a) California
15. b) Unconstitutional
16. c) The Day the Earth Stood Still
17. c) Rock 'n' Roll
18. c) Ford
19. d) Andy Warhol (Note: while the exact date of Warhol's statement is debated, it became iconic of his perspective and the evolving media landscape of the mid-20th century.)
20. c) Katharine Hepburn
21. a) Hal March
22. d) Vertigo
23. b) Bobby Darin
24. d) Mayberry
25. d) Singin' in the Rain
26. c) 12 Angry Men

27. c) John F. Kennedy
28. d) Trick question, this quote is from "Toy Story" (1995)
29. d) Space Patrol
30. b) The Everly Brothers
31. c) Vertigo
32. b) Global domination
33. d) A Streetcar Named Desire
34. c) Bill Haley & His Comets
35. b) Battleship
36. b) Jeopardy!
37. c) Paul McCartney
38. d) Ben-Hur
39. b) Twister (Note: While the patent was filed in the early 60s, it's a reflection of the innovative game design of the era.)
40. d) North by Northwest
41. c) Perez Prado
42. c) Scrabble
43. d) Ben-Hur
44. a) Frank Sinatra
45. b) Building a mousetrap
46. d) Love Me Tender
47. b) Mambo
48. c) The Day the Earth Stood Still
49. c) Clue (or Cluedo)
50. c) Singin' in the Rain
51. c) Alan Ladd
52. c) Yo-yo

53. d) Patti Page
54. c) The Ten Commandments
55. c) Life
56. a) Hawaii
57. a) Jack Kerouac
58. d) McDonald's
59. c) Barbie Doll
60. c) Charles Lindbergh
61. b) Aluminum
62. c) Dwight D. Eisenhower
63. c) Mustang
64. c) Romper Room
65. b) Microwave oven
66. b) Poodle skirt
67. d) Willie Mays
68. c) Jonas Salk
69. d) Marilyn Monroe
70. c) Rock 'n' Roll
71. a) Electric kettle
72. a) Color television
73. c) Petticoats
74. b) Steve McQueen
75. d) I Love Lucy
76. b) Egypt
77. b) Ray Bradbury
78. b) Pompadour
79. a) Jitterbug
80. a) The Beatniks
81. b) The Beatles

82. c) The Sound of Music
83. b) Jenga
84. a) Audrey Hepburn
85. b) The Animals
86. c) Twister
87. a) Tom Jones
88. c) The Middle East
89. c) Monopoly
90. c) Spaghetti Western
91. a) The Supremes
92. b) Hula Hoop
93. a) Sean Connery
94. a) The Doors
95. b) Operation
96. a) Dustin Hoffman
97. d) God Only Knows
98. c) Clue
99. a) Audrey Hepburn
100. d) Apollo 11 Mission
101. d) Psycho
102. b) Woodstock
103. c) Mary Quant
104. c) San Francisco
105. c) One Flew Over the Cuckoo's Nest
106. d) United States
107. c) Lite-Brite
108. a) The Rolling Stones
109. d) The Twist
110. b) Lyndon B. Johnson

111. c) England
112. c) Star Trek
113. d) Bedrock
114. c) Martin Luther King Jr.'s March on Washington speech
115. d) The Pixie
116. c) The Sound of Music
117. b) The Beach Boys
118. d) The Feminine Mystique
119. a) Rubik's Cube
120. c) Love
121. d) The Watusi
122. b) The Jetsons
123. c) Mary Poppins
124. c) Bikini
125. c) Peace and love
126. c) Mini Cooper
127. b) The 5th Dimension
128. b) Nuclear disarmament
129. b) Butch Cassidy and the Sundance Kid
130. d) John Glenn
131. c) Muhammad Ali
132. d) I Dream of Jeannie
133. c) Leslie Gore
134. c) Human Be-In
135. c) Moon Watch Party
136. b) Ed Sullivan
137. b) The Mamas & the Papas
138. b) Elizabeth Montgomery

139. c) Landing a man on the Moon
140. c) Louis Armstrong
141. b) The Twist
142. d) Yellow Submarine
143. c) Woodstock
144. b) Dr. No
145. b) Roger Bannister
146. a) Lite-Brite
147. b) Tupperware Parties
148. a) The Sound of Music
149. d) Music
150. b) The Flintstones
151. b) Civil Rights Act
152. c) Bell-bottoms
153. b) M&Ms
154. d) Star Trek
155. d) Walt Disney World
156. b) 23rd Century
157. d) Neil Armstrong
158. b) Raga
159. b) Summer of Love
160. b) Bewitched
161. a) Fleetwood Mac
162. d) Willy Wonka & the Chocolate Factory
163. b) Jimmy Connors
164. c) Mazda RX-7
165. b) Jeopardy!
166. c) The Brady Bunch
167. d) The French Connection

168. b) Army hospital
169. c) The Carpenters
170. d) Butterfly collars
171. a) Gerald Ford
172. a) Jaws
173. d) Pink Floyd
174. c) Yo-Yo
175. b) Alex Haley
176. b) Grease
177. c) Atari
178. c) Lite-Brite
179. a) Charlie's Angels
180. b) Little House on the Prairie
181. a) Don McLean
182. a) Gloria Gaynor
183. c) Hip thrusts
184. c) Funny Girl
185. c) Elvis Presley
186. a) Kinte
187. b) Fat Albert
188. d) Star Wars
189. c) Mark Spitz
190. a) 1970
191. c) Gilligan's Island
192. c) Roberta Flack
193. c) Sesame Street
194. c) Sylvester Stallone
195. a) Bell-bottoms
196. d) Montreal

197. d) The Hustle
198. b) The X-Files (Note: The X-Files began in the 1990s, not the 1970s.)
199. c) E.T. the Extra-Terrestrial
200. b) Tennis
201. a) 1970
202. c) Hee Haw
203. c) Apple
204. c) The Jetsons
205. d) Bobby Fischer
206. b) Actually a rock
207. b) The Eagles
208. c) Mork & Mindy
209. c) VHS
210. a) Roy Lichtenstein
211. c) Illuminated pegs
212. c) Taxi Driver
213. b) Byte
214. d) Studio 54
215. c) Faye Dunaway
216. b) Mr. Potato Head
217. b) Bell-bottoms
218. c) ThingMaker
219. b) Disco
220. b) Taxi
221. a) Perm
222. b) Monopoly
223. c) Smokey and the Bandit
224. a) Rod Stewart

225. c) Isle of Wight
226. b) Mary Tyler Moore Show
227. c) 7-Up
228. b) Digital numbers
229. c) Columbo
230. d) Whac-A-Mole
231. b) Bee Gees
232. c) Camera
233. b) Bee Gees
234. a) The Love Boat
235. a) Saturday Night Fever
236. c) Martina Navratilova
237. c) New York City
238. a) Chevrolet Impala
239. a) Bell-bottom pants
240. c) YMCA
241. b) Knight Rider
242. c) Madonna
243. c) NES (Nintendo Entertainment System)
244. c) Risky Business
245. c) Jazzercise
246. b) Paul Fusco (voice of ALF)
247. d) Back to the Future
248. b) Rubik's Cube
249. c) R.E.M.
250. a) Jelly sandals
251. d) Andy Warhol
252. c) Pac-Man
253. c) The Tanners ("Full House")

254. b) The Richard Simmons Show
255. b) Cheers
256. d) Transformers
257. d) The Breakfast Club
258. c) Tina Turner
259. c) Frogger
260. a) Mohawk
261. b) Family Ties
262. c) ThunderCats
263. c) Sony
264. d) DeLorean DMC-12
265. c) Macarena (Note: The song became a hit in the 90s, but it was initially released in the 80s.)
266. c) Footloose
267. a) Creepy Crawlers
268. b) Prince
269. a) Mouse Trap
270. c) MTV
271. d) Jane Fonda
272. b) To tell time
273. b) Pound Puppies
274. b) E.T. the Extra-Terrestrial
275. c) Matthew Broderick
276. c) Pepsi
277. d) MECC
278. b) Leg warmers
279. c) The Police
280. c) Macintosh
281. b) Dallas

282. c) He-Man and the Masters of the Universe
283. c) LeVar Burton
284. c) Lite-Brite
285. c) "Don't Stop Believing"
286. b) A skateboard
287. b) Cabbage Patch Kids
288. c) Duran Duran
289. c) Galaga
290. c) Magnum P.I.
291. c) New Coke
292. c) The Goonies
293. b) Donkey Kong
294. a) "Thriller"
295. b) Space Hopper
296. b) Cheers
297. a) Simon
298. c) Madonna
299. b) Mork
300. c) Listen to music on the go
301. d) Mr. Potato Head
302. a) Jazzercise
303. b) Labyrinth
304. c) Take On Me
305. a) Baywatch
306. d) Fireball Island
307. c) General Hospital
308. d) Shrinky Dinks
309. a) Designing Women
310. d) Converse

311. a) Lego
312. b) The Tanners
313. c) Teenage Mutant Ninja Turtles
314. a) Cabbage Patch Kids
315. c) Supermarket Sweep
316. c) Guns N' Roses
317. d) Family Ties
318. a) Electric Slide
319. a) Magnum, P.I.
320. c) Robot Dance
321. c) Friends
322. d) Tamagotchi
323. b) Magic 8-Ball
324. c) Macarena
325. c) Barney
326. d) Platform shoes
327. a) Will Smith
328. c) Rugrats
329. b) The Lion King
330. a) Backstreet Boys
331. c) PlayStation
332. c) Aqua Ranger
333. d) Water Snake
334. b) Spirograph
335. d) Jessie
336. c) Legends of the Hidden Temple
337. a) Tetris
338. d) Compact Disc (CD) player
339. a) Cheers (Note: "Cheers" actually premiered

in the 1980s, but it continued and was popular
in the early '90s.)
340. d) Beanie Babies
341. c) Sabrina the Teenage Witch
342. c) Tropical Fruit Fever
343. a) Michael Jordan
344. c) Spain
345. c) Kodak
346. a) Hanson
347. d) Rugrats
348. a) Guess Who?
349. d) Sam Neill
350. a) Glow Worm
351. a) Hook
352. b) Urkel
353. a) Animorphs
354. c) Oasis
355. d) Larry the Llama
356. d) Sega Genesis
357. c) Pogo Ball
358. b) Cookie Crisp
359. b) Saved by the Bell
360. d) Stretch Armstrong
361. c) "Beautiful Life" - Ace of Base
362. a) Extremely wide legs
363. b) Friends
364. c) Barcelona
365. a) Will Smith
366. c) LEGO

367. b) Julia Roberts
368. a) No Doubt
369. c) Google
370. d) Crystal Pepsi
371. c) Goosebumps
372. c) Giga Pets
373. c) The Little Mermaid
374. c) Madonna
375. c) Niles
376. c) Apple
377. c) Buffy the Vampire Slayer
378. c) Spice Girls
379. c) Japan
380. a) Cast Away
381. b) Furbies
382. d) Sony
383. d) The Proposal
384. c) Los Del Rio
385. c) AOL Instant Messenger (AIM)
386. b) J.K. Rowling
387. d) Michael Jordan
388. b) Malibu Beach
389. b) The Lion King
390. b) Creepy Crawlers
391. a) Slap Bracelets
392. d) Clippy
393. d) Rugrats
394. c) Apple
395. b) Prince

396. a) X-Files
397. a) Will Smith
398. d) The Hunchback of Notre Dame
399. b) NewsRadio
400. d) Jumanji

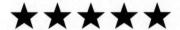

SHARE YOUR THOUGHTS!

Dear Reader,

Have you finished the book? We'd love to hear your take on it! Please consider leaving an honest review because your feedback guides other readers and helps us grow.

How to Leave a Review

Scan the QR code, which will take you to the review page.

Your voice matters. Lend it to the conversation and help shape future reads!

Thank you.

Printed in Great Britain
by Amazon

37721338R00071